Life ⁻

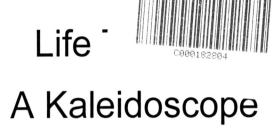

C000182804

A Kaleidoscope

Experiences Of Scotopic Sensitivity
Syndrome – Memoirs Of Visual
Fragmentation

Paul Isaacs & James Billett

chipmunkapublishing
the mental health & autism publisher

Published by

Chipmunkapublishing

PO Box 6872

Brentwood

Essex CM13 1ZT

United Kingdom

http://www.chipmunkapublishing.com

ISBN   978-1-84991-937-1

Chipmunkapublishing   gratefully   acknowledge   the support of Arts Council England.

Index

All subject names have been subject to change

Many Thanks to James Billet & Susan Rowling

Introduction James Billett Irlen Consultant

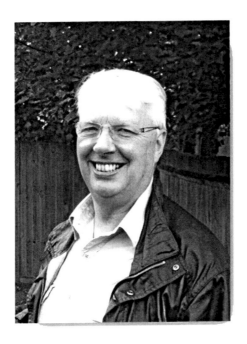

© **James Billett 2012**

The wonder of the World Wide Web brings many people together. However, Paul first approached Irlen Central England not through an email enquiry but by a phone call, he needed to establish for himself what was likely to happen during an assessment. This is not unusual since people need the reassurance of a voice and manner before committing themselves to a particular service. During the conversation it was immediately apparent how thoughtful, self-aware, meticulous and precise Paul is.

There is no need for me to describe what happened during our working session together as Paul will do this later.

After seeing Paul what I did say to the family when I got home was "I have just met a walking textbook for Irlen and autism". This isn't because of the symptoms which Paul has, these are familiar in themselves and as a pattern. A textbook is an instruction book, a source of knowledge and information; this is Paul. The suffering he has experienced and described so vividly in "Living Through The Haze" is a template of experience and hope. Hope, that a more enlightened and diagnostic approach could spare others from such experiences. Experience in offering a path of future progress.

What is so different about working with ASD? Only after working with special needs children for twenty years and with the Irlen Institute for ten years would I have the confidence to work with Autism. Only through the experience of Donna Williams would I have the knowledge of how to help clients with ASD.

This is not because autistic persons are different from others, the opposite, autistic people have exactly the same response to stimuli and communication as each of us. What is so different is that the response, the sensation, the fear, the joy are more intense, heightened, stimulating and ultimately frightening. There is also the sense of being trapped, held forever in a faulty response to the world. This response can be seen by others as a pathological condition.

I discovered the work of Helen Irlen 1989, out of sheer desperation. At the time I was trying to teach adolescents to read and looking for anything to help. I got the name Irlen by dialing a free phone line available as a part of dyslexia awareness week. It was the name only, then it was just a drag through directory enquires spelling the word any way I could until a phone number was found. I didn't find Helen Irlen through advice from established educational or medical advice and neither did Paul. It was an LEA Special Needs Advisor who told me that the best things in Special Education are private as they offer flexibility. The history of change and progress is through committed individuals. I am both privileged and pleased to be able to help Paul with this book.

Introduction Paul - Autistic Author, Trainer & Speaker

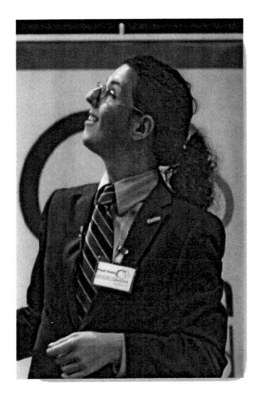

© Isaacs/Autism Oxford

My name is Paul Isaacs. I was diagnosed with High Functioning Autism in 2010 at the age of 24. For many years, through my speeches, I had talked about my problems with processing visual images, understanding depth, recognising objects, people, and faces and having problems with processing words and numbers.

Through my years as a non-verbal child with severe autism I appeared deaf and blind, not seeming to understand my surroundings and not hearing sounds. My parents were very concerned about this as documented in *Living through the Haze,* my autobiography.

In the summer of 2012 I found out about Irlen Central UK and James Billett, who is a specialist in Irlen Syndrome (Scotopic Sensitivity Syndrome), working with clients whose conditions include Autism, Asperger's Syndrome, ADD, ADHD, Dyspraxia, Dyslexia, Dyscalculia & Learning Disabilities. James has worked with Helen Irlen since 1990, meeting and helping people of all ages and difficulties in both the public and private sector.

James remembers meeting Donna Williams at the Irlen Clinic in which her filters were first diagnosed. He recalls how Donna was not only able to describe so clearly her own perceptual experiences and the impact of the prescribed Irlen filters but how Donna was so sensitive and gifted so as to transfer and translate her experiences and make them so relevant for others.

James is a caring person and the consultation was a wonderful positive experience. He employs a person centred approach, he let me go at my own pace and would discuss the process in a way in which I understood. He talked with me about my dyslexia, dyscalculia, semantic agnosia (meaning blindness), simultagnosia (object blindness), prosopagnosia (face blindness) and body disconnectedness, all of which he was able to confirm. It was a wonderful experience and the realisation of how different my visual processing was until I found the right lenses. It was a moving experience of clarity and understanding which I will never forget. James has seen this reaction many times and he sincerely believes in helping others and this came across in this highly professional consultation.

To James, I thank you! ;-)

Prosopagnosia

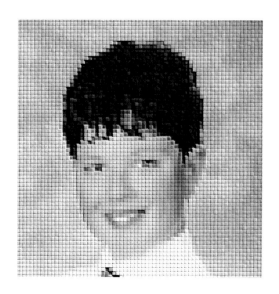

I can't process faces. It's a difficult task as the picture above suggests. The face is a combination of small pieces of complex information. I can only process one piece at a time, as I don't have a visual memory. I can't retain the small pieces of information in a manner which is collective and whole. This means that a face is far too fragmented to process as a whole piece of information. Meaning that even if I have met the person once before, I will not retain that visual information. The only reference I have had for people is their hair because that makes up the largest coherent whole that isn't as difficult as the face.

For many years people would say *"hello"* to me and I would respond back not knowing if I knew them or not. This can be very difficult at times because it can cause a lot social embarrassment. I have had many incidents when people have had conversations with me and I have no idea whom I'm talking to.

I have learned over time, through a realisation that I'm having problems with faces, to recognise the voice of the person and use that as a "marker" for knowing, processing and remembering that person.

Boris has a life alone, an educated adult living in his parent's house, spending hours on the computer. Boris was aware that he must be on the ASD spectrum but living in Turkey was unable to obtain diagnosis. Having emailed James and completing the Irlen questionnaires James, who had already booked a holiday with his wife in Olu Deniz, took his case of Irlen lenses with him. Boris took a 17 hour bus ride to the Resort, James did the assessment during the afternoon finishing in time for Boris to catch the bus back home. When the correct colours were established Boris said "I can see that you have a nose now." How strange it must be to live in a world where faces mean nothing.

Simultagnosia

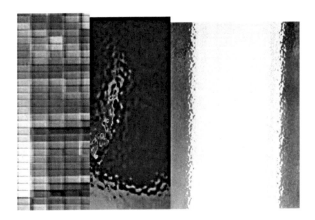

As the title of the book suggests life is very much like a kaleidoscope in terms of visual bombardment. The Kaleidoscope is both beautiful and stark, amazing yet awful, all at once. This is the paradox.

I have created and manipulated images above to give you a representation of what I see and how I process and can manage visual information, piece by piece and one part at a time. It's tiring and stressful, causing panic attacks, fatigue, headaches and in extreme cases dizziness and nausea.

I have problems with depth perception and see things in a matte 2D image. As I move my head and body every image is switching and processing on a flat plane with no understanding of depth, not knowing how far things are away in foreground and background. Life is very much like a painting of a blocky minimalist nature.

The paradox is that some colours and sounds I love, getting attracted to them and wanting them close by me and close to my eyes. This has been something I have done for many years with paints as a young child. I would spread them across the paper with my bare hands, moulding coloured play dough over and over. I was also fascinated by water, its formlessness and how it changes into different colours. As an adult some of these things still calm me when I'm stressed and in meltdown. Certain fabrics (felts, leathers and soft materials) still calm me. I purchased this colourful magic "wand" from a supermarket; the colours spin green and orange and I can play with it for hours, laughing and stimming to my heart's content.

Stimming is such a part of ASD, the pleasure and the pain of sensory overload. The good thing is the wonder and sense of colour and life in the world. But, like so many aspects of Autism, James sees the sadness of parents. How can it feel to watch your seven year old son, Declan, sitting alone in the lounge and spending a large part of the day searching for imperfections and scratches on CD's.

Semantic Agnosia

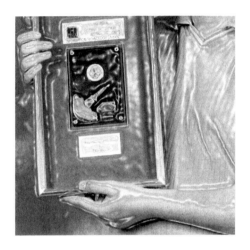

Donna Williams explains about the hands being the "eyes" of people who have 'meaning blindness'. I agree with her; my hands are where my sensory receptors are and I can remember liking my hands and feet to be free to run and touch and feel my surroundings. I would mouth, lick, sniff, tap, rub my body and face around my visual surroundings trying to get a basic "map" of where I was and what I was touching and feeling. Understanding came much later in my development;

however this is still a problem for me. This will explain why my parents thought I was blind and had a visual problem that was to do with my eyes. It was not a physical problem with the organ (my eyes) itself but the way in which my brain was, and still does, process visual information and how I gauge surroundings. As ever, it is Donna Williams who related Autism and sensory deprivation, by watching blind children at play and realising that was how she related to the environment.

As I have got older these things are still very much a part of me. However, I feel because of the need for social conformity and to lessen the exploitation and bullying I have had to "switch off" these needs. However, where I feel most comfortable in the safe haven of my home, I still do these behaviours because they're a part of me and I don't feel ashamed of them. My parents have obviously been the most aware of this aspect of me as they accepted from an early age that this was 'me'.

James stresses the need for ASD children to find a security in the environment. Home for most people is a nest, a space apart from the world. For a child with ASD the home is a bewildering series of interlinking never ending spaces. James once invited a single mother and her severely non-verbal 3 year old to come to the UK for recognition and support that was not available in their own country. His most vivid memory of Timandra is not of her running around the house like a steam train but of finding her asleep in a cot in the baby room. Laying against the four sides of the cot gave her a sense of security. A dog sleeping for the night will generally prefer for its back to be touching something. We all live in a world of constant visual over stimulation; touch is still a primal need.

Dyslexia

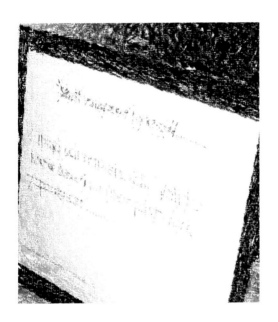

Dyslexia was apparent during my school years. I always seemed to be "behind" in development in terms of reading and writing. As I got older many problems still persisted such as mixing words up and letters, with words either mixing up, adding or taking out letters, reducing the flow of my writing. I also still have problems with punctuation which is really an issue when writing but I have help with this aspect. The way in which I "see" words is a jumble and it's like a misty fog over the letters which makes them hard to read and understand.

I have problems with handwriting which causes fatigue in my fingers, hands, wrist and arm. I was also getting so tired writing I felt like I was holding my breath as I wrote because of the sheer amount of concentration I had to put into every word and sentence. This caused further problems with comprehension.

That is why I'm really thankful that I can touch type because even though mistakes are made they can be changed and rewritten. I think schools and teachers should really work to a student's own style. From my past experience I would say that if a pupil finds writing an issue, other alternatives should be made as it would show a better representation of the pupil's potential and skills.

Dyscalculia

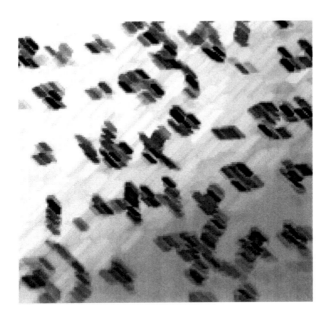

Numbers for me are just as difficult in processing as words. I remember trying to recite my times tables wondering how this would help me retain information which I felt was the real issue with maths. I couldn't process the formulas on the board; I would write them, look at them and try to understand the task and sequence which I couldn't because it was this mash of lines, numbers and symbols which made no sense. If I didn't understand the question there was no way that I was going to get the answer!

The problem with words was exported over to numbers and many different methods were tried although none of them worked because the teachers weren't getting to the "core" of the problem and where my difficulties were coming from. To them it looked like defiance or even laziness.

Again it caused fatigue in my arms, wrist, hand and fingers so concentration was affected. I remember day dreaming a lot in my maths classes because help or assistance wasn't there in the context of what I needed, and I suspect others in the class had similar problems too.

Words and numbers move. Harriott is a friend and colleague of James who is an Assessor of Dyslexia for Universities in the East Midlands. One question she always asks students is *"What is happening to this page?"* and *"how do you feel when you look at the words?"* If only teachers had asked this question long before. Dorothy is just completing her degree in Photography. Dorothy is diagnosed with mild Dyslexia and mild Dyspraxia, 2012.

"I have always had problems with reading and writing. School was quite hard; I was always in the lower classes. That's why I worked myself up from foundation level. I used to have to go for reading lessons at 8 o'clock in the morning. My pictures were always better than my writing. I was told to type it up and stick it in a sketch pad. If I am walking the floor moves, and if I have to put a key in the lock it is hard, the door frame moves. I get dizzy in the road when I am driving and hit the kerb. A lot of the course is practical and I enjoy the research. My grades have gone up from 40-50 in Year 1 to 60+ now. I have been coming to the workshops and this has helped me because before the tutors could not read or understand my writing. My grades have gone up since then. Reading? Not even for ten minutes! I would love to sit there and be able to read and get more information."

For Dyslexic clients James uses key indicators to eliminate text distortions:

This is Dorothy talking about the effect of her Irlen filters:

Wall Chart:

Before: *"It hurts. They are starting to blur stop if I focus on one letter I can see 3. The rest of the letters are just grey I can't tell you what they are."*

After: *"It's clear. I could tell you 9 or 10 letters it is so clear…. It's a different world isn't it, that's an amazing thing."*

Typical number and letter confusions, pdq 385 etc:

Before: *"They get all blurry."*

After: *"They are dead, totally clear."*

Page of text:

Before: *"I can't read that at all!"*

After: *"I can read that now."*

One word on the text book page:

Before: *"I have to stare at it and take my time with it otherwise it is just so hard to read."*

After: *"It is clear absolutely. I can't tell you how amazing it is."*

	Before	With Irlen filters
Wall Chart	*"It hurts. They are starting to blur stop if I focus on one letter I can see 3. The rest of the letters are just grey I can't tell you what they are."*	*"It's clear. I could tell you 9 or 10 letters it is so clear…. It's a different world isn't it, that's an amazing thing."*
Typical letter confusions.	*"They get all blurry."*	*"They are dead, totally clear."*

Page of dense text	*"I have to stare at it and take my time with it otherwise it is just so hard to read."*	*"It is clear, absolutely. I can't tell you how amazing it is."*
One word within a page of dense text	*"I can't read that at all!"*	*"I can read that now."*

In many occupations numbers are more important than words. Rachael is training to be a nurse. Henry is a member of the Armed Forces.

356996583	Before	With Irlen filters
Rachael	*"The numbers merge into one."*	*"That is the first time I have realised that they are in a row. Because you are not spending so much energy focusing on it you can see what is there."*
Henry	*"It's just… you can't look at it."*	*"It's okay you can look across the lines and read them."*

To achieve this result James worked with Dorothy in two separate sessions, a total time of around three hours. So please remember this if you are thinking that obtaining the correct combination of coloured filters is a quick optical fix.

The normal length of time to establish the correct colours is around two hours.

James was invited to work on the West Coast of Ireland, the parents of ASD children had set up a school themselves. Having worked with Eamon, a severe verbal ASD boy, James asked his mother how the optician had arrived at the necessary optical prescription, Eamon's mother replied *"he doesn't let him into the shop, Eamon sits in the car with his seatbelt and the optician passes lenses through the window."*

For ASD clients James prefers to see a person in their own home, somewhere that they are comfortable with and aware, in their own way, of familiar objects and the make up of the room. In order to be a non threatening adult James may sit still and be quiet, just having a cup of tea and talking with the mother of the ASD child, at the same time watching and learning about the child until it is the time to begin. However before the session the family will have completed the detailed Irlen Autism questionnaire. This questionnaire not only details specific visual indicators of heightened or reduced sensory response but places them within the context of the complex pattern of related autistic behaviours. James insists upon parental or carer involvement in the tinting session; he asks, who else would know their child better? Louise brought her Asperger's son to the UK specifically for a consultation. Louise: *"James, if you had not spoken a word during the session I would have known how much the lenses helped Derek by the expression of his face first and that I have never heard him read like that in his life before."* The effect of the filters is both immediate and cumulative.

Everything coming together

When I saw James for the appointment, maybe I wasn't fully prepared for what I was going to experience, it was a moment of clarity and things coming together! I was amazed it was something for over 26 years I had just "lived with", thinking that many people had the same issue as me.

As I have documented above the various processing problems, agnosias and learning difficulties that compact and make up my ASD, what I was pleased about is that the Irlen lenses had a multi-layered approach to how I perceived things.

As I walked around my sitting room things seemed and were more "connected", I felt connected in my environment, after years in which I felt so detached and "foreign". I looked at objects I found hard to process, such as a small tree in my back garden. I said to James "oh, it has a middle bit" - what I was trying to say was that the connectivity from the leaves, branches and the trunk of the tree were all connected.

I looked at James when he came in; he was in "pieces" and my eyes strained, focused and re-focused trying to get the "totality" and wholeness of whom I was seeing. Luckily I am very perceptive and have good "sensing" skills. James is excellent and professional. He has been working with people with ASDs for many years, has a calm person-centred approach which made me able to communicate and open up to him. Pieces of his body came together like a jigsaw. I was seeing a whole person and it wasn't overwhelming (at least in a visual sense, inside I was very overwhelmed). I processed his face not just seeing an "eye" or a "tooth" or a "mouth" but a vast interconnectivity of how the face is formed and processed. This was in the first 10 – 15 minutes of putting on the correct lenses. It was instant of course but I was taken aback at what I was "seeing" for the first time in a very long time.

It also helped with my dyslexia and dyscalculia. I was quicker at processing the words and reading them out. I was also processing long strands of numbers which, like the letters and words, didn't seem muddled, jumbled up or "hazed".

It was an amazing experience; for the first time I saw clarity and the world in a different way. Let's list what these Irlen lenses have helped me with.

- Prosopagnosia (face blindness)
- Simultagnosia (object blindness)
- Semantic agnosia (meaning blindness)
- Visual – Verbal agnosia (written comprehension)
- Dyslexia
- Dyscalculia

Through the diagnostic assessment with James all these things he understood, recognised and will implement into the written diagnosis of Scotopic Sensitivity Syndrome, that is the multi-layered affect it has had on my processing. It has helped me with not just one thing but yet another and another! For the first time my eyes felt "free" and not under any stress or pain.

I could not have got these from an optician's because they deal with the physical organ that is the eyes and not the processing behind the eyes (the brain). I was diagnosed with short sightedness when I was around 5 years old. I wore awful glasses which caused me pain and discomfort because, as James put it, they "magnified" the problems. In recent years I have worn them less and less; they are still in the house, broken, old and dirty, they bear no use.

I could not have acquired these lenses anywhere else because opticians do not specialise in the problems which I was experiencing. Maybe what could happen is the opticians should be trained to recognise SSS/ILS and be able to refer the individual onto a person like James who is qualified and able to make a diagnostic assessment.

Here are some examples of Irlen Central UK's work and how it has helped people like myself.

Why Irlen Works: Mythbusting

James

Back in 1993 the Local Authority Educational Psychologist for the school area in which I taught assured me that coloured lenses couldn't possibly work as her friend was an optician and he had told her so. Within three years the same optician was providing coloured lenses and now lots of opticians offer to provide treatment for 'visual stress'. This is but a micro example of the initial reaction of the medical and optical profession to Helen Irlen's first research paper delivered in 1983 to the American Psychological Association.

Although Helen Irlen began her revolutionary treatment method by using a range of coloured overlays to cover a page as she listened to clients, she soon learned that distortions also happen on wall charts and posters. This is why Helen developed a range of coloured lenses.

Later it was Autistic clients who explained that, for them, problems are not confined to text - everything moves.

An Aspergers' boy asked *"what colours are you going to choose for me?"* I replied, *"Thomas, you will be choosing the colours, I am just helping you."*

If you wear glasses think about what happens when you have your eyes tested. In order to choose glasses, you keep looking through different ones chosen by the optician comparing them until you are both certain that things are as clear as they can be; this is called the "matched pairs" method. This is exactly what happens when you have the Irlen lens evaluation but unlike the standard optical tests things are much more complicated because we are not actually working with the eyes but the brain's response to confusing visual stimulation. Irlen Syndrome is not an optical condition but something, like dyslexia, which is happening deep inside the brain with the pathways that transmit messages from the eyes to the visual cortex. Independent MRI and Spect scans confirm that there is an abnormal pattern of information processing. Since distortions are not confined to the printed page, they also vary in different lighting conditions. The Irlen evaluation will include near and far distance, natural light, fluorescent light, and your balance. By the end of the session everything should be clear and still, and believe it or not, whatever colour your glasses are, the page will still look white for you, and nothing will look a different colour to what it should, this is because the lenses filter such small bands of incoming light they do not affect your vision. Whatever colours you choose will be because you have looked through the lenses and chosen them yourself, what you have seen and felt is exactly what you will get, made up for you in California. Once you have them the glasses can be worn all day, every day and at night time too. Remember, your basic problem is being sensitive to light.

People who go to an optician will have a very different experience of choosing colours. Basically you will put your head inside a machine and choose the particular colour you like best as coloured lights shine on a page. The shade you prefer (then, that is it) will be made up into glasses for you. The session will last around 20 to 30 minutes. The shade will be three times darker than Irlen colours [independent research University of Modena]. You have chosen a reflection (light coming off a surface) and not a refraction (light coming through a lens). Coloured glasses from opticians usually come with a warning that the colours may distort vision and colour sense and should not be worn in some situations. An Optician told me a story about one of his clients – A frightened ten year old boy came home from school telling his mother that his eyes had been bleeding all day. The Optician said *"I told the mother this was quite normal. He needs dark red glasses and his brain would soon get used to it."* Let's think some more. You have gone to the opticians because you are sensitive to light and this triggers, amongst other things, movement on the page, headaches, problems with a VDU, and/ or fluorescent lighting. Now, have you chosen your colour in a darkened or windowless room? Did you actually look through the lenses and see how you felt, if you could tolerate fluorescents, watch a VDU or was it later when they had been made up that you were first able to assess their efficiency? If this seems a bit of a problem, one dyslexia/coloured lens specialist works by Kinesiology, lifting up the client's arm to test reactions to each coloured lens.

Here are some people who have been to Irlen Central England talking about their earlier experiences with opticians and colour.

"I never really noticed the difference with them; I don't think that they are right to be fair. Sheffield sent me there. I don't think the optician knew what they were doing really. I wasn't in there very long, I was only there about 10 min."

"I can wear them for a two-hour block. When I take them off everything has a green tint to it. When I am wearing them the page is a pink red, like a sunset. My colour sense is distorted, everything goes to a reddy pink, which is the reason I only wear them when I am reading. For reading I can see 10 fonts but my eyes jump around and there is this peach effect. I do try to wear them as sunglasses as it makes me more comfortable and stops me from squinting. The lenses reduce the symptoms but I am unable to see a white board or a video with them on so if I am in a lecture or a classroom I have to keep pushing them off my eyes and onto my head to be able to see things. Then I wonder where they are."

"I made the stupid mistake last year of going to an optician for coloured lenses. My seizures went up to twice a day and I had permanent headaches. I lasted five weeks and it cost me £600. They gave me pink glasses; it took ten or fifteen minutes and a green and yellow overlay. The overlay was a cheap plastic film. It never occurred that having pink glasses would make my seizures worse."

"The Cerium lenses haven't done what they promised. They tested my reading rate and said it went up 15% but it is unrealistic to wear them all day. You can't function with them."

"I picked overlays for the glasses. I am on my 3rd colour... These glasses are weird, everything that is lower down is closer than it should be; everything is. Your feet look really close and your head looks really far away. The side of a square will be coming towards me; it is most noticeable when I use my laptop. It doesn't happen with my glasses on. I told my opticians when I got them and they just said 'see how it goes'. I have got used to it but it is not right. "

Sarah "The last time we went was 2 years ago, the gentleman lifted up Callum's arms, we weren't in there very long, he was determined that Colin needed two different colours, green and purple; after that everything fell apart." Colin is Asperger's, "I wore the purple glasses on Tuesday and Thursdays, the green glasses on Monday Wednesday and Friday."

Here are some words that confuse people:

Scotopic Sensitivity Syndrome, this is the first term Helen Irlen used and it is still true as it means light sensitivity syndrome.

Irlen Syndrome is a visual-perceptual disorder which is neurologically-based, affecting the visual cortex and linked to a transient or magnocellular deficit in the pathways of the brain.

Irlen Syndrome is Disability S100909/02 according to the 2010 Equality Act.

See also 'The Safeguarding Vulnerable Groups Act 2006 (Miscellaneous Provisions) Order 2009 No. 1797' where Irlen Syndrome is listed, amongst others, as a disability.

Meares-Irlen Syndrome has been a name used by others to link their work to Helen Irlen.

'Visual stress' is a descriptive term for symptoms which are neither a visual or medical condition in order to overcome trademark infringements from using the Irlen name since opticians and organizations other than Irlen Clinics have no connection with Helen Irlen or the Irlen

Lightning Source UK Ltd.
Milton Keynes UK
UKOW040943150313

207690UK00001B/9/P